UNLOCKING

THE

EROTIC CAPABILITY

OF

CHOCOLATE

An Enthralling Expedition Through Exotic Nature and Joy.

Aldis O. Sherwood

1 | Aldis O. Sherwood

TABLE OF CONTENTS

INTRODUCTION

It was a Wednesday, the day I'd been looking forward to. John and I picked today for our evening date. John was a guy I met through a mutual, we've been going out for 4 months, and despite that, I'm giddy for tonight's date. Why? because we are trying out the chocolate version of romance. John has allergies so it took us a while to discuss the products and if he feels comfortable with it. So, this is me looking forward to our chocolate night. As a chocolatier, it's not a new process but I have to be sure of my partner's comfort. I lifted my legs a little before spreading them wide by the edge of the bed. I leaned back but propped myself up by my elbows. John was at the edge of the bed, the lust in his eyes was evident, and so was mine. His eyes traveled to my clit covered in melted chocolate, he blinked once, then twice, his pupils were dilating at the sight of my dripping clit. Everything about him says he couldn't wait to latch his tongue on my clit, and so he did. A gasp escaped my lips as I looked at him from the rearview, his boner was rock-hard. He ran his tongue across my knees, licking off the chocolate while also running his fingers across my skin getting closer to my sweet spot, I moaned. He saw my inviting clit glistening with chocolate and let out a groan, it was musky, enough to let out the juices my vagina has been withholding, but I didn't. I needed to know if I could outlast him, I needed to see who releases first. He moved up his hand but refused to touch me which made me whimper. He smiled. I groaned internally. He thrust his middle finger through my clit which made a groan escape from me. He moved his finger through my warm, wet, and sweet sex in a circular motion which made my juices flow out. I was dripping off my cum and chocolate. I looked up to see John licking his soaked hand. I wanted more, and from his look and I

5 | Aldis O. Sherwood

know he also wanted more. He fell to his knees and used his fingers to spread my pussy lips before thrusting his tongue into me. I yelled in ecstasy which made him aroused more than he already was. Faster, I yelled, he stopped to scoop more chocolate on my clit while his fingers were doing wonders to my right nipple.

It was a cloud nine.

Barely anything on the planet have interested and tempted people across societies and time like the luscious appeal of chocolate. Past its liberal flavor and soothing properties, chocolate holds a secretive appeal that has been related to want, enthusiasm, and romance for a long time. From old civilizations crediting incredible powers to the cacao bean to current darlings savoring its enticing characteristics, chocolate has established its place as an immortal aphrodisiac that mesmerizes the senses and lights the blazes of intimacy.

In this exploration, we venture on a captivating journey through the verifiable, social, and mental perspectives that entwine chocolate and exotic nature. The expedition will uncover the antiquated Mayans and Aztecs' confidence in the heavenly properties of cacao and its part in sacred rites. We will navigate the European Renaissance, where chocolate turned into a portrayal of extravagance and enticement, gracing the courts of respectability, and encouraging romantic connections. The fusion of chocolate with various ingredients and flavors offers a plethora of possibilities, allowing couples to indulge in a symphony of taste, touch, and aroma, creating a feast for the senses.

Besides, we will dive into contemporary practices where chocolate remains an essential piece of heartfelt gestures and personal encounters. From trading boxes of chocolates on Valentine's Day to enjoying delectable chocolate pastries during candlelit suppers, we will observe how chocolate keeps on bringing out enthusiasm and friendship in present-day connections.

As we dive further into opening the sexual capability of chocolate, we will explore how it tends to be integrated into cocktails, treats, and tactile encounters to boost intimate experiences. The combination of chocolate with different ingredients and flavors offers excess potential outcomes, permitting couples to enjoy an ensemble of taste, touch, and aroma, making a banquet for the senses.

All through this exploration, we will uncover the scientific premise that adds to chocolate's status as an aphrodisiac, digging into the mixtures that trigger sensations of joy, prosperity, and excitement when consumed. Also, we will encounter stories of passion and allure, where chocolate has been a charming instrument in arousing desire and connecting hearts.

8 | Unlocking the Erotic Capability of Chocolate

Eventually, this enrapturing expedition will feature how chocolate's sensual characteristics reach out a long past its taste and smell. By embracing chocolate's extravagance with care and imagination, couples can set out on a journey of revelation, delight, and closeness. Whether commemorating an exceptional event or trying to reignite the enthusiasm in their relationship, unlocking the sensual capability of chocolate guarantees a captivating and remarkable experience that rises above time and culture. Therefore, prepare to be charmed by the enchanting powers of chocolate as we dive further into the specialty of unwrapping its suggestive charm — a tour that vows to stimulate the senses and stir the inner passion.

CHAPTER ONE

Significance of Sexual Health and Delight

Sexual health and pleasure are necessary parts of overall well-being and quality of life, enveloping physical, emotional, and mental aspects. Fostering a positive and satisfying sexual experience is fundamental, as it allots to different parts of an individual's prosperity, relationships, and all-around satisfaction. Exploring the importance of sexual well-being and delight requires a complete assessment of its different aspects.

Genuinely, immersing in regular sexual action has been related to various medical advantages. Scientific research recommend that sexual action improves cardiovascular well-being, boosts the immune system, and improves better sleep. Additionally, the discharge of endorphins during sexual activity functions as a natural pain reliever, lessening anxiety and improving all-around sense of well-being. A satisfying sexual life can contribute to a better reproductive system. For all kinds of people, regular sexual activity can help to strengthen the reproductive organs and decrease the risk of certain ailments. For women, sexual activity can strengthen pelvic floor muscles, which can be advantageous during child labor and later in life.

Notwithstanding the physical advantages, sexual pleasure likewise plays a significant part in emotional and psychological well-being. Intimate connections and sexual experiences can prompt increased feelings of intimacy, trust, and emotional closeness with lovers. A delightful sexual life encourages a feeling of satisfaction and bliss, adding to positive psychological wellness. Moreover, experiencing pleasure during sexual activities can help with decreasing sensations of uneasiness, stress, and depression, functioning as a natural stress reliever, and improving emotional balance.

Additionally, embracing sexual well-being and delight enables people to become more sensitive to their bodies and wants. This self-awareness encourages a better understanding of individual preferences and limits, prompting further improved communication and mutual satisfaction with partners. Feeling confident about one's sexuality and welcoming pleasure without embarrassment or remorse can boost confidence and body certainty. This confidence stretches out past the room and decidedly influences different parts of life, including relationships and professional endeavors.

Sexual well-being and pleasure are essential parts of a fulfilling and delightful life. Focusing on and fostering one's sexual well-being offers a heap of advantages, including physical well-being, emotional well-being, and healthier relationships. By embracing a positive and empowering method to deal with sexual well-being and pleasure, people can lead more joyful, healthier, and more connected lives. It is fundamental to improve open discussions, reduce stigma, and develop an environment that enables everybody to embrace their sexuality with certainty, respect, and delight.

Role Of Aphrodisiac in Enhancing Sexual Experiences

Since ancient times, aphrodisiacs have been part of human culture and history. They are thought to have mystical properties that heighten desire, passion, and ecstasy during sexual relations. These compounds, whether they be organic or synthetic, are supposed to increase arousal, heighten the sexual experience, and boost libido. Aphrodisiacs' significance in increasing sexual experiences is a topic of intrigue and curiosity with people from different cultures searching for their special way to stoke desire.

Aphrodisiacs have been linked to sexual desire and delight since the dawn of human civilization. For their purported aphrodisiac qualities, some foods, herbs, and organic materials have been adored throughout history. To have more intense sexual encounters, various societies have embraced a wide variety of aphrodisiacs, from oysters and figs in ancient Rome to saffron and honey in ancient Persia. These notions weren't just folklore; ceremonies and traditions involving fertility, love, and romance frequently included aphrodisiacs in ancient societies. These substances were also alluring in literature, where poets and authors constantly referred to their capacity to arouse passion and sensuality.

Aphrodisiacs' potency also stems from the psychological effects they have. An individual's perspective of their sexual encounter can be affected by their simple belief in these substances' power. This psychological phenomenon has the potential to increase sexual arousal, build anticipation, and promote self-assurance.

14 | Unlocking the Erotic Capability of Chocolate

Aphrodisiacs may occasionally function by calming people down and lowering performance anxiety. Alcohol and other drugs can lessen inhibitions and promote intimacy in a more relaxed and open environment, improving the overall sexual experience.

Some aphrodisiacs have physiological effects that can improve sexual encounters. For instance, the molecules in chocolate can boost the production of endorphins, or "feel-good" hormones, causing a feeling of pleasure and happiness. Some aphrodisiacs, like ginseng and maca root, are said to increase energy and blood flow, which could perhaps heighten arousal and sexual performance. Additionally, diets high in specific minerals, such as zinc and vitamin E, might promote hormone production and reproductive health, which may have an impact on sexual desire.

Aphrodisiacs can help couples connect emotionally and promote communication by introducing them to a

15 | Aldis O. Sherwood

shared experience. A deeper emotional connection might result when both people are willing to explore aphrodisiacs jointly because it can spark excitement and adventure. Talking about preferences, tasting new cuisines, or experimenting with scents and flavors may all be enjoyable ways to strengthen relationships. The willingness to experiment with aphrodisiacs can increase intimacy and trust, resulting in a more satisfying sexual experience.

As a result, there is a complicated interplay between cultural beliefs, psychological affects, physiological effects, communication, and sensory stimulation in the use of aphrodisiacs in increasing sexual encounters. Whether or not aphrodisiacs' effects are supported by science or are merely a placebo, their attraction continues to draw those who want to arouse desire and passion in their private interactions.

Accepting the investigation of aphrodisiacs, whether they take the shape of foods, smells, or experiences, may give intimate relationships an exciting new dimension and promote a closer bond between lovers. But it's critical to utilize them with open communication, respect for personal preferences, and an emphasis on shared enjoyment and consent. As with any facet of sexual activity, the true magic is found in the sincere understanding and connection between lovers, which fosters a loving and safe environment for shared intimacy.

CHAPTER TWO

The Historical Connection of Chocolate To Romance.

The story of the relationship that chocolate has historically had with romance and desire spans eras, nations, and civilizations. Over the course of human history, chocolate has been venerated as an indication of passion and pleasure, from its discovery and consumption by prehistoric Mesoamerican civilizations to its introduction in Europe during the Renaissance.

The cacao tree (Theobroma cacao), which is the source of chocolate, first appeared in Mesoamerica in antiquity. Cacao was seen as a divine gift and connected to vitality and fertility by the Maya and Aztec cultures. Chocolate beverages were only consumed during sacred rituals and ceremonies, and cacao beans were employed as currency. These ancient cultures thought that eating cacao increased desire and provided spiritual vitality, strengthening the relationships between lovers.

Early in the 16th century, the Spanish explorer Hernán Cortés was essential in bringing chocolate to Europe. Cortés brought the unusual drink back to Spain after seeing the adoration the Aztecs had for cacao. Initially, only the Spanish aristocracy and kings were known to love chocolate. The European nobles were captivated by its alluring flavor and the rumor that it had aphrodisiac qualities, which led to a chocolate frenzy among the aristocracy.

The connection between chocolate and romance and desire grew during the Renaissance. The velvety, sweet drink, which was served in European royal courts, came to represent opulence and sensuality.

Chocolate houses gained popularity as gathering places during the 17th and 18th centuries, especially in England

Similar to modern coffee shops, these places offered a place for people to congregate, interact, and indulge in chocolate-flavored beverages. Chocolate shops are favored hangouts for courting couples because of their inviting ambiance that encourages romantic meetings.

As it gained popularity, chocolate started to be given as preferred by lovers. Giving chocolate as a gesture of love has come to be associated with romance, especially on holidays like Valentine's Day. Even now, the tradition of exchanging chocolate boxes as a symbol of love and desire is still practiced.

The reputation of chocolate as an aphrodisiac has scientific justification in addition to its historical significance. Numerous substances found in chocolate can cause the discharge of neurotransmitters linked to delight and well-being. One such substance is phenylethylamine, also known as the "love chemical," which causes sensations of exhilaration and enthusiasm.

Also included in chocolate is anandamide, also referred to as the "bliss molecule." A neurotransmitter called anandamide attaches to receptors in the brain and causes feelings of joy and contentment. Another ingredient in chocolate called theobromine functions as a mild stimulant and may help to increase energy and alertness.

The romantic association between chocolate and desire still exists today. When sharing a decadent chocolate dessert over a candlelit meal or playing around with chocolate body paint, couples frequently include chocolate in their intimate interactions. The sensuality of chocolate is still valued as a way to deepen intimacy and pleasure in love partnerships.

While many cultures associate chocolate with passion and desire, it is crucial to keep in mind that the symbolism and rituals associated with chocolate can differ greatly from one culture to another. For instance,

Valentine's Day in Japan is a day on which women present chocolates to men, and there is a separate holiday known as "White Day" on which men return the favor.

The tale of intrigue and interest around the historical link between chocolate and desire, and romance is fascinating. The allure of chocolate as an aphrodisiac and a symbol of desire has persisted throughout history, from its sacred Mesoamerican origins to its passage through European courts and modern rituals. Due to its sensual delights, cultural importance, and scientifically proven aphrodisiac effects, chocolate remains a popular indulgence during private moments. As couples eat decadent chocolate delicacies to commemorate their love or exchange boxes of chocolates on important occasions, chocolate's reputation as a sign of adoration and desire remains unwavering. The fascinating association between chocolate and romance endures, making it a delightful and enduring tradition in the world of love and desire, whether in literature, art, or real-life rituals.

CHAPTER THREE

The Role of Chocolate in Romance And Desire

The fascinating history of chocolate's relationship to passion and desire spans eras, nations, and civilizations. Due to its attractiveness, this delicious dessert has frequently been linked to wants, delight, and indulgence, making it a representation of sensuality and passion in a variety of contexts. Chocolate's sensual power has had a significant impact on how people express desire and closeness, from its place in love stories to how it is depicted in art.

The custom of giving and receiving chocolates as a sign of love and affection first originated during the Victorian era. Couples frequently exchange boxes of chocolates, especially on Valentine's Day and other special occasions. Giving chocolates to a close friend or family member represented sweetness, adoration, and desire. As a common courtship gift, admirers would present the person they were courting with a box of chocolates as a loving gesture. This custom is still widely used today, and chocolates are still a traditional symbol of love and devotion.

The sensual appeal of chocolate has also captured artists, who use it in their creations to arouse desire and sensuality. Paintings of chocolate-covered pastries or fruits can suggest indulgence and temptation. The glossy surface of chocolate can reflect light and shadow to produce a seductive visual impression that appeals to the viewer's senses. Additionally, the act of eating chocolate can be portrayed in art as an intimate time between two people, highlighting the sensuous connection that the food can evoke. Couples eating chocolate together or sharing it in paintings and sculptures represent their closeness on an emotional and physical level.

Chocolate has been cleverly marketed in the world of marketing as a treat that piques desire and pleasure. Advertisements for chocolate frequently employ seductive language and sensual imagery to seduce customers. Chocolate consumption is portrayed as a pleasant experience that intensifies the senses and arouses positive emotions. Brands market their chocolate goods as perfect presents for memorable events or acts of love by associating them with ideas of sensuality and romance. Chocolate's association with desire and passion in contemporary society has been largely reinforced by the sensuality portrayed in its marketing.

The sensual appeal of chocolate comes from more than just cultural connotations; it also comes from the sensory delights it provides. A holistic experience that includes touch, smell, and taste can be created by the flavor and texture of chocolate. A luxurious and sensual experience can be created by the silky texture that melts in the mouth, the diverse taste notes that range from sweet to bitter, and the lovely perfume.

Chocolate frequently occupies a prominent position in actual loving gestures. Giving someone you care about a box of chocolates might be perceived as a concrete way to show them how much you care. Sharing chocolate can represent the sharing of love and intimacy because the sweetness of the chocolate is sometimes compared to the sweetness of relationships. Couples also regularly use chocolate in their romantic date evenings, utilizing it to heighten the sensual and pleasurable experience. Couples discover ways to satisfy their senses and celebrate their relationship with this favorite indulgence, from sultry candlelit dinners with chocolate-based pastries to amusing activities utilizing chocolate.

The sensual seduction of chocolate has also sparked a variety of activities and occasions dedicated to the treat.

27 | Aldis O. Sherwood

A joyous and delicious ambiance that heightens the senses is frequently created by chocolate festivals, where visitors can try a variety of chocolate delicacies. Additionally, those looking for novel and sensory experiences can take chocolate-making lessons or receive spa treatments with a chocolate theme.

CHAPTER FOUR

How Chocolate Stimulates the Brain's Pleasure Center

Scientists and chocolate lovers alike have been fascinated by chocolate's capacity to elicit positive emotions. A complex interplay between sensory perception, physiological processes, and psychological responses all plays a part in the undeniable pleasure that chocolate induces in the brain.

The brain's pleasure center, a complex network of neuronal connections predominantly controlled by the discharge of neurotransmitters like dopamine, serotonin, and endorphins, is at the center of this relationship. These molecules are essential for controlling the state of mind, emotions, and pleasure response.

Not only are you savoring the flavor of the chocolate, but you are also igniting a neuronal symphony.

Dopamine is released in the brain after eating chocolate. With each bite, dopamine sometimes referred to as the brain's "reward molecule," increases. Your brain is giving you a mental pat on the back, which makes you feel good and makes you want to indulge more. This neurochemical reaction is similar to the joyful feelings one could have after partaking in delightful activities like taking part in physical activity, listening to music, or spending time with friends and family. Another neurotransmitter, serotonin, joins the fun and adds to the comfort and well-being you experience when eating chocolate. Serotonin levels may momentarily rise after eating chocolate, which can boost feelings of well-being and relaxation. This may help to explain why many people use chocolate as a comfort meal when they're under stress or going through a difficult moment.

Theobromine is one of the essential ingredients in chocolate that gives it its satisfying benefits.

Theobromine is 'The Underestimated Player'. It is a less-publicized component of chocolate; it functions as a mild stimulant. It acts as the conductor of this cognitive orchestra, enhancing attentiveness and boosting blood flow to the brain. This may be the reason why a box of chocolate might give you a mental lift in the middle of the afternoon. In cacao, the main component of chocolate, there is a natural substance called theobromine.

Additionally, eating chocolate takes you on a sensory adventure. Multiple senses are stimulated by the interaction of its silky texture, wonderful scent, and rich flavors. This sensory extravaganza stimulates pleasure-related brain areas, enhancing our delight. The distinct fusion of taste, fragrance, and texture in chocolate adds to the overall delightful experience. The brain's reward circuits are tightly related to our sensory impressions.

The enjoyment of chocolate is not just a physiological phenomenon; psychology also plays a role in it. The long tradition of celebration and excess surrounding chocolate has woven a web of favorable associations in our minds. Do you recall how wonderful it was to get a box of chocolates on a particular day? Our enjoyment of chocolate is enhanced by these recollections, making it a favorite comfort food.

Although chocolate has undeniably enjoyable benefits, it's important to consume it carefully. As your brain becomes accustomed to the elevated levels of dopamine, overindulgence might result in declining effects. Consuming chocolate in moderation makes sure you never run out of its delightful charm.

A dance of neurotransmitters, sensory perceptions, and psychological associations is involved in chocolate's ability to activate the pleasure area of the brain. Our brains produce a symphony of pleasure because of theobromine's effect as well as the discharge of dopamine and serotonin. As you enjoy your next chocolate treat, keep in mind the fascinating interaction between science and pleasure that occurs with each mouthful.

CHAPTER FIVE

Dark Chocolate- The Powerhouse of Pleasure

One of life's greatest pleasures, dark chocolate is frequently referred to as the "powerhouse of pleasure." Its fascination goes beyond its mouthwatering flavor, combining a symphony of tastes, sensations, and healthy advantages that enthrall the senses and the body.

A treasure trove of tastes that make every bite enjoyable can be found behind its velvety shell. The star of the show is the dark chocolate's high cocoa content, which provides a range of flavors from bitter to sweet with hints of earthiness and even a trace of fruity acidity. Each indulgence becomes a sensory adventure thanks to this intricate taste dance.

Consuming dark chocolate is a sensory adventure that involves more than just the taste buds. Its opulently silky texture melts on the tongue, and its earthy richness-like perfume builds expectation. These sensory signals interact to produce an experience that is equally focused on pleasing the palate and the senses.

Beyond the immediate pleasures it provides, dark chocolate contains a variety of bioactive substances that may be beneficial to health. Strong antioxidants called flavonoids, which are present in cocoa, fight oxidative stress while enhancing general health. These substances maintain a healthy circulation of blood, may lower the risk of heart disease, and have been related to improved heart health. Even if these results are encouraging, it's crucial to consider dark chocolate as a part of a healthy diet.

Another aspect of dark chocolate's attraction is its capacity to elevate mood. A natural stimulant called theobromine helps to elevate mood and increase attentiveness. A further layer of pleasure, comparable

37 | Aldis O. Sherwood

to the ecstasy experienced from physical exertion, is added by the endorphin release brought on by eating dark chocolate.

Choosing varieties of dark chocolate with a greater cocoa content—ideally 70% or more—ensures a more effective dose of its health-promoting ingredients, allowing you to enjoy the treat to the fullest. However, since dark chocolate is high in calories, moderation is still a must.

The flexibility of dark chocolate is also evident in culinary artworks, where it enhances anything from sweets to savory foods. Because of its bittersweet flavor, it pairs well with wines, cheeses, and fruits to offer a variety of palate-pleasing partnering options.

As a result, dark chocolate goes beyond its status as a simple sweet treat and is a "powerhouse of pleasure." A complete experience that entices the senses and nourishes the body is created by the interaction of flavors, sensations, and potential health benefits. Keep in mind that the delights of dark chocolate are an appreciation of culinary brilliance and a monument to the amazing potential of nature's riches as you appreciate its depths.

White Chocolate- Debunking Myths and Exploring Its Potential.

White chocolate is a fascinating topic that has been the focus of numerous culinary arguments and misunderstandings. We may discover the hidden gems that make white chocolate a special and adaptable ingredient with uses well beyond the dessert plate by eliminating myths and exploring its immense possibilities.

Myth 1: White chocolate isn't "real" chocolate: White chocolate isn't considered "real" chocolate because it doesn't contain any cocoa solids. However, it's crucial to recognize that cocoa butter, the decadent fat derived from cocoa beans, is where white chocolate gets its flavor. This pricey component helps give white chocolate its distinctive flavor and silky texture.

Myth 2: Nutritional Deficiency: Even while white chocolate doesn't have the same number of antioxidants as its darker siblings, it still has beneficial ingredients. Healthy monounsaturated fats, calcium, and phosphorus that support bone health are all present in cocoa butter. White chocolate has some nutritional benefits despite not being an antioxidant powerhouse.

Myth 3: Cloyingly Sweet: White chocolate is frequently criticized for being too sweet and bland by critics. However, this perception can be imaginatively used to complement and harmonize other flavors. The natural sweetness of white chocolate can be skillfully paired with sour fruits, zesty citrus, or aromatic herbs to create elegant and tasteful culinary combinations.

Myth 4: Limited Use: White chocolate may be used for a variety of things outside just sweets. It works well in both savory and sweet meals thanks to its mild flavor and creamy texture. Its capacity to surprise and amaze extends to everything from spiced sauces and creamy soups to white chocolate-infused spaghetti.

Beyond the Kitchen: The world of white chocolate is not limited to the kitchen. The moisturizing qualities of cocoa butter have been used by the cosmetic and skincare sectors, demonstrating the potential of white chocolate in lotions, moisturizers, and lip balms. Beauty rituals can become sensual experiences thanks to their silky smoothness and gentle aroma.

The potential of white chocolate in beverages is broadened. White chocolate-based syrups could be used in craft cocktails and specialty coffees to give a decadent flavor and eye-catching appeal. Think of a luscious hot chocolate with white chocolate undertones or a creamy white chocolate mocha.

Busting preconceptions about white chocolate reveals a world of culinary inventiveness and originality. Although unique to dark chocolate, its distinctive makeup provides a blank canvas for exquisite flavors and creative mixes. Beyond flavor, the potential of white chocolate permeates the fields of skincare, beverages, and other areas. By embracing the actual essence of white chocolate, we unlock doors to a world where culinary craftsmanship and practical applications coexist, enabling us to explore, discover, and savor newly discovered delights.

Milk Chocolate - Finding the Balance Between Creaminess and Desire.

Milk chocolate is a classic treat that expertly manages to satisfy both the urge for unquenchable yearning and the exquisite creaminess that tantalizes the senses. Milk chocolate is an enchanted treat with far-reaching ramifications because of the harmonious interaction between texture and temptation, which creates a sensory symphony that sings to the heart and palate.

The luxurious smoothness of milk chocolate is where its seduction first begins. Milk solids, cocoa butter, and cocoa solids work together to create a smooth, velvety texture that melts on the tongue with ease. Due to the flawless blending of the components, milk chocolate has a seductive texture that gently embraces the senses.

The delicate sweetness of milk chocolate is essential to its charm. The addition of milk solids creates a subtle sweetness that melds well with the subtle cocoa aromas. This harmony keeps the sweetness from overpowering the complex flavors of the chocolate, resulting in a satisfying and nuanced sensory experience.

Milk chocolate carries feelings and memories in addition to being delicious. Each bite can take us back to happy and nostalgic times. A milk chocolate bar's appearance might bring back childhood memories of peeling foil, and its flavor elicits sentiments of familiarity and closeness. Milk chocolate becomes more than just a treat thanks to this emotional resonance; it becomes a means of reliving special occasions.

Milk chocolate is a work of art that goes beyond simple ingestion. Chefs use this ingredient's adaptability to create a variety of mouth-watering dishes. The versatility of milk chocolate and its capacity to work well with a variety of ingredients are demonstrated by the luscious truffles, velvety ganaches, and subtle pastries. The ability of milk chocolate to amplify and heighten flavors is demonstrated in this culinary symphony.

The appeal of milk chocolate extends to beverages as well. The balance of milk chocolate is best exemplified by the draw of hot chocolate with its creamy and foamy appeal. The drink's frothiness, which is finished with a sprinkling of cocoa, embodies the harmonic union of creaminess and desire and invites us to embrace comfort and contentment.

However, moderation is still crucial when pursuing excess. Milk chocolate's velvety charm and overwhelming desire can easily result in overindulgence. Using restraint not only makes it easier to appreciate each bite but also helps to keep the beautiful atmosphere around for other occasions.

Milk chocolate is the ultimate culinary invention. Its adaptability allows for a variety of savory and sweet treats, making it a blank canvas for creativity. Milk chocolate improves every creation, from desserts to drinks, by fusing creaminess and desire into an orchestration of tastes and feelings.

The flawless harmony between creaminess and desire that milk chocolate achieves is what makes it so alluring. A transcendent experience is produced by its luxurious texture, subtle sweetness, and emotional resonance. We engage in a dance of pleasure and longing as we taste its velvety caress and welcome the longing it awakens. Because it forever entwines creaminess and desire in an ensemble of exquisite delight, milk chocolate's timeless attraction serves as a gentle reminder that life is most enjoyed when we achieve a balance between our yearnings and our senses.

CHAPTER SIX

Sensual Tasting - Exploring Chocolate as An Exciting Foreplay Experience.

I smelt the room before I entered, Chocolates. I walked in, and scented candles which made the room dimly lighted are scattered all around. A soft melody playing in the background, and the room is filled with an intoxicating smell of different flavors of chocolate. On the table lie different flavors of melted chocolate with strawberries, nuts, and bananas. John urged me to try his arranged delicacies. It's not a new dessert to me as a chocolatier, but it's John's first time preparing it without my guidance. He wanted to surprise me, and he did. I dipped a strawberry into the melted dark chocolate. A taste of it heightened my senses. A moan escaped my lips when John's hand reached out to me pulling me closer to him. His lips touched mine and I felt my whole body on fire reacting to his touch. Our *lips moved in perfect sync, our bodies melding together as it was supposed to be. We stopped for a while to feed each other fruits dipped in melted chocolate. At the last bite, his hands closely encircled my waist, and he pulled me tight against his chest. It's going to be a long night with our bodies speaking the language they understand better.*

Chocolate is an appealing partner for sensual tasting, an intimate assessment that thrills the senses. Couples who explore the alluring realm of the sensual chocolate tasting set off on an extraordinary voyage of intimacy and discovery. This luxurious encounter sparks desire, encourages emotional ties, and elevates chocolate to a powerful catalyst for sparking romance.

Imagine a room that is dimly lit, with relaxing melodies playing in the background, and a variety of chocolates placed in front of you. The creative prelude that precedes sensual tasting is a symphony of anticipation that awakens the senses. The visual enticement of several chocolate varieties, each with a unique tale to tell, creates the ideal environment for the upcoming sensory investigation.

The adventure begins with the inhaling of the enticing aroma of chocolate. An alluring aroma of earthiness, floral undertones, and the promise of the sumptuous flavors to come fills the space as the chocolate is brought closer. Arousing the sense of smell builds up anticipation and prepares the body for the event to come.

The feel of chocolate between the fingertips invites physical interaction. When the surface is examined, a variety of textures are revealed, ranging from the silky smoothness of milk chocolate to the somewhat rough embrace of dark chocolate. An intimate dance develops between the tactile exploration and the moment the chocolate melts on the tongue.

While enjoying the chocolate, a crucial moment occurs. The palate is met with a variety of flavors that develop gradually, starting with sweetness and moving on to cocoa's complexity and the flavors' mild harmonious interaction. Couples discuss their thoughts on the symphony of flavors that inspire feelings and encourage discourse. Of course, combining chocolate with other flavors that match it can enhance the sensuous experience even more. Try pairings like sea salt, roasted nuts, citrus zest, or even a taste of coffee or red wine. The flavors of chocolate are emphasized and increased by the other components in these combinations, which can produce harmonious sensory experiences. Discover how the interactions of the flavors of sweet, salty, bitter, and acidic dance on your taste buds.

A shared adventure of vulnerability and intimacy is created by sensual tasting, which goes beyond the act of consuming. The sharing of chocolate treats develops into an act of mutual submission to the feelings elicited. Couples become immersed in a private conversation that strengthens their relationship beyond only the physical. The act of sensual tasting chocolate can arouse and pique desire. The sensory investigation sharpens perception and heightens need. As a result of their shared experience, their passion is stoked, creating the ideal environment for a more passionate and rewarding romantic encounter.

Sensual taste serves as an emotional connection's catalyst beyond the momentary pleasures. Couples dive into their desires, tastes, and shared memories as they discover the subtleties of chocolate. The encounter turns into a voyage of personal growth and mutual understanding, establishing the basis of their connection.

Oral sensations can also be enhanced with chocolate. Couples can have a special and enjoyable experience by including chocolate in their foreplay. The use of edible massage oils or body creams with chocolate flavors, for instance, can enhance the sensuous massage experience while also providing a delectable flavor. To improve oral sex, lovers can also experiment with chocolate-flavored lubricants. For both parties engaged, the combination of the sweet, chocolatey taste and personal acts can be immensely enjoyable and exciting.

Homemade body and massage oils can be prepared with chocolate. Couples can make their massage oils or body butter. Butter are infused with chocolate by melting cocoa butter and adding aromatic oils. A delicious and enjoyable massage can be created by sensually applying the warm and silky texture of cocoa

53 | Aldis O. Sherwood

oil to the skin. Additionally, the fragrance of chocolate has a calming impact on the psyche, which contributes to the development of a cozy and private atmosphere. Couples' overall pleasure and connection can be increased by massaging each other with oils that have been infused with chocolate.

Chocolate and ice cubes can also be combined for individuals who like to play with temperature. Couples can make tiny chocolate disks or shapes that can be applied to various erogenous zones by melting chocolate and letting it cool just a bit. It might be tempting and provocative to experience the contrast between the ice's coldness and the warmth of the chocolate. To create a special and enjoyable sensation, partners might alternately use their tongues to lick and suck the chocolate off one another's body.

Chocolate can cause sensory deprivation and eagerness for individuals seeking more daring experiences.

Couples can explore their senses by blindfolding one another and utilizing chocolate as a surprise element. A thrilling and sexy sensation can be created by the suspense of not knowing where the chocolate will be applied next together with the enjoyment of its taste and texture. The excitation and anticipation generated by this type of sensory play can increase pleasure and satisfaction.

It is crucial to buy high-quality, food-grade chocolate that is suitable for consumption while using chocolate in the bedroom. Use of chocolate that has added sugars or artificial tastes should be avoided because they may irritate or create pain. Before including chocolate or any other food in your personal moments, it's crucial to discuss with your spouse, set boundaries, and get their approval. It's also critical to be aware of any dietary restrictions or food allergies that can prevent you from using particular chocolate products.

The experience of sensual tasting with chocolate transcends the sense of taste. It is a waypoint to greater intimacy, an investigation of desire, and a celebration of connection. Couples enhance their romantic experiences to new heights as they embrace the symphony of flavors, textures, and feelings that chocolate brings. The ritual of sensual tasting turns into a treasured reminder that passion and connection are deeply woven into the fabric of the senses. Couples learn the power of shared delight through the luxury of chocolate, turning ordinary moments into unforgettable memories.

Chocolate Body Paint - Adding a Delicious Twist to Erotic Exploration.

The act of intimacy is transformed into a seductive and delectable adventure by chocolate body paint, a decadent union of taste and touch. This lavish artwork gives the field of erotic exploration a delicious and sensuous twist, producing a painting of desire that invites lovers to set off on a voyage of deeper connection, playful exploration, and unforgettable intimacy.

Imagine a setting where a chocolate body paint palette is waiting, soft music is playing, and candlelight creates a cozy atmosphere. A seductive blend of pleasure and cuisine, this encounter starts as an invitation to indulge. A trail of expectation is left on the skin by the paint's silky texture, intensifying all the sensations. As partners transform into painters and create their most private works of art using chocolate body paint, the body becomes a canvas for desire. Every application is a whisper of longing, every stroke a caress. Each brushstroke is a promise of the passion to come as the act of painting and the act of receiving merge into a dance of sensual beauty.

It is a trip of flavor and teasing to use chocolate body paint. With each touch, partners experience the chocolate's richness, blending the anticipation of touch with the flavor. The experience is both luxurious and invigorating as the sweet tones of chocolate blend with the heady sensations. The application of chocolate body paint goes beyond the physical act and promotes a closer relationship between partners. A strong emotional connection is facilitated by the vulnerability of exposing one's body, the closeness of touch, and the exchange of glances. Touch and eye contact between partners create a language of passion that words are unable to express.

Chocolate body paint, a powerful aphrodisiac, ignites romance by encouraging sensory exploration. Desire catches fire like a slow-burning flame as partners enjoy the pleasurable process of tasting and stroking one another. A beautiful dance of longing and pleasure is created by the interaction between the sweetness of chocolate and the electrifying emotions it induces. Using chocolate body paint results in more than just the instant feelings; it also leaves behind lifelong memories. A treasured moment that forms a part of a couple's romantic journey is when they disclose a private secret. The lingering impression of that sensual encounter serves as a reminder of their strong bond and close-knit playfulness.

Finally, the tapestry of romantic discovery is enhanced by the tasty and enticing addition of chocolate body paint. Couples are invited to embark on a journey that awakens the senses, strengthens emotional ties, and arouses libido. Partners create a shared experience that honors the art of seduction and the pleasures of intimacy as they savor the physical pleasure, relish in the taste, and create sensual art on one other's bodies. Chocolate body paint becomes a tasty and entertaining instrument that turns genuine connections into priceless memories.

Sensory Stimulation - Incorporating Chocolate into Sensual Massage and Touch.

When sensuous massage and touch are combined with chocolate, sensory excitement is elevated to new heights. This irresistible pairing produces a decadent sensation that stimulates the senses, encourages connection, and elevates everyday experiences into remarkable journeys of pleasure. Couples embark on a journey that celebrates the interaction of taste, touch, and emotion by mixing chocolate with sensual massage, which helps to strengthen their bond in a truly special and exquisite way.

Along with its mouthwatering flavor, chocolate also has a rich scent and a velvety texture that add to its attractiveness. The use of chocolate in sensual massage creates a feast for the senses. The aroma of the chocolate-infused oil permeates the room as it is warmed between palms, setting a seductive mood. A deeper connection is facilitated by the oil's silky glide over the skin, which heightens tactile sensations and engages touch in a sensual dance. Massage oils with chocolate flavoring are created by combining cocoa butter or beans with a carrier oil, such as almond or jojoba. The warm and smooth texture of the chocolate oil when applied to the skin during a massage induces a profound sense of relaxation and pleasure. Additionally, the fragrance of chocolate has a relaxing impact on the mind, which helps to lower tension and increase feelings of wellbeing. The body and mind are left feeling renewed and invigorated as a result of the massage strokes and the chocolate-infused oil's delectable mix.

Additionally, using chocolate during a sensual massage has the amazing ability to melt away barriers and restraints. Couples who are frequently reluctant to discuss their wishes find themselves enclosed in a cocoon of mutual vulnerability. Applying chocolate-infused oil transforms into a surrendering and trusting gesture, opening the door for real emotional and physical connection.

The addition of chocolate to sensual massage adds a fun tease factor. The skill of delicately tasting the chocolate while tracing designs on each other's skin can be practiced by partners. When taste and touch combine, the feelings are amplified and produce a deep, satisfying symphony. The fact that chocolate is temperature-sensitive makes the experience more unexpected. When chocolate-infused oil is applied to the skin, the warmth of the palms and body heat heighten the sensations. Sensitivity is increased by the contrast between the cooler oil and the warmer touch, which results in a seductive dance of hot and cold that awakens the senses.

Sensual massage, in turn, is a type of non-verbal communication, a language of touch that expresses feelings, aspirations, and intentions. The inclusion of chocolate improves this language, enabling lovers to communicate their love and longing in a special and delectable way. A common communication that transcends words is created with each brush, caress, and hand press. A sensuous massage filled with chocolate is more than just a physical act; it's an intensely private encounter that creates a strong bond between partners. Massages are given and received as acts of devotion, as an expression of love and caring.

63 | Aldis O. Sherwood

Partners establish a sacred environment where they are totally present and attentive to the sensations and feelings that arise.

The combination of sensual massage and chocolate has the potential to lead to pleasure. Taste, touch, and closeness together provide an inflow of pleasure that elevates states of arousal. Partners explore erogenous zones and ignite passion in a way that transcends the limits of the physical world as they travel the geography of desire.

A sensory harmony that commemorates pleasure, connection, and shared indulgence is created when chocolate and sensual massage are combined. The use of chocolate-infused oil adds a variety of sensations that intensify the experience of touch, from the mouthwatering aroma to the delicious taste. As they partake in this intimate rite, partners negotiate a terrain of desire and emotional kinship, developing a deeper tie that goes beyond the ordinary. A beautiful method of communication, a celebration of the senses, and a voyage of shared ecstasy, sensual massage with chocolate leaves an everlasting impression on the fabric of intimacy.

CHAPTER SEVEN

Decadent Dessert - Indulging in Chocolate's Delights for An Intimate Evening.

There is a delicious secret in the world of quiet evenings: the rich dessert. This indulgence, a symphony of flavors and feelings, is a thrilling ballet of the senses and a celebration of chocolate's alluring seduction, which transforms a regular evening into an amazing trip of intimacy.

Dessert is not just an afterthought; it is a mouthwatering introduction that teases the pleasures to come. Imagine a table set with flickering candles, soothing music filling the air, and the star of the show being a masterfully prepared dessert. The stage is set for an intimate exploration that warrants not only gastronomic delight but also a reawakening of libido. A sensory masterpiece emerges as the dessert is exposed. There are gasps of anticipation as the aroma of chocolate fills the space. The subtle crunch of a chocolate shell giving way to a luscious interior, layers of flavor sensations blending in perfect ecstasy—the first bite is an orchestration of sensations and flavors.

Sharing a sumptuous dessert is a symbol of mutual indulgence and an intimate sharing that spans the distance between two souls. In the pursuit of pleasure, partners become co-conspirators, with each mouthful igniting a shared memory. An unseen bond formed by their knowing glances and mischievous smiles conveys their love for one another. The attraction of chocolate as an aphrodisiac gives the evening an additional dimension of magic. Partners are engulfed in a wave of intensified sensations with each bite. The same substances that provide pleasure, phenylethylamine and serotonin, also contribute to a feeling of euphoria, fostering a cozy and intimate environment.

Chocolate-based sweets are a mainstay of sensual cuisine. These treats, which range from silky smooth chocolate mousse to molten lava cakes dripping with warm chocolate ganache, are made to arouse the senses and stoke passion. A thick and silky chocolate dessert can be a romantic experience in and of itself. A sumptuous and sensual moment can be enjoyed alone as a form of self-indulgence or shared between lovers thanks to the dessert's rich flavors, silky texture, and powerful flavors that engulf the palate.

Together, enjoying a delectable dessert makes enduring memories that stick in the heart and mind. Long after the final morsel has been enjoyed, the remembrance of that shared moment serves as a touchstone for reigniting romance. The dessert begins to represent their relationship and the love and desire they have for one another.

A night of indulgence is more than simply a sensory treat; it's a chance to strengthen relationships. Partners enjoy each other's company while conversing freely and without interruption. The dessert serves as a trigger, encouraging an atmosphere of vulnerability and openness.

Finally, the sumptuous dessert serves as a vehicle for shared intimacy, a spark for romance, and a blank canvas for partners to express their aspirations. Couples go on an explorational, connecting, and adorational journey as they indulge in the pleasures of chocolate. Their relationship's tapestry is forever changed when the flavors of chocolate meld with the flavors of their love. A testament to the ability of shared indulgence to foster closeness, the opulent dessert becomes a celebration of the senses, an ode to passion, and a celebration of the senses.

69 | Aldis O. Sherwood

Chocolate Covered Fruits - Combining Natural Aphrodisiacs for Enhanced Pleasure.

Chocolate-covered fruits stand out as a seductive liaison between nature's aphrodisiacs amid the subtle interplay of flavor and desire, opening the door for an enchanting exploration of sensuality. Couples are invited to participate in a symphony of flavor, texture, and intimacy by this exquisite convergence, which immerses them in a moment that transcends the ordinary and turns mundane moments into extraordinary voyages of passion.

A seductive aphrodisiac alchemy is produced when certain fruits and chocolate are combined. The natural antioxidants present in fruits like strawberries and figs help to promote a general sensation of well-being as the phenylethylamine contained in chocolate travels through the veins, causing feelings of pleasure and bliss. This flavorful combination serves as a culinary trigger for heightened perception and deeper connection.

Imagine a dish filled with delectable fruits like juicy oranges, plump figs, luscious peaches, and mangoes, all covered in a luxurious layer of chocolate. Just the sight awakens the senses, tantalizing the taste and captivating the eyes. A sensory ballet that speaks directly to the tactile senses is sparked by the first bite, which is a symphony of sensations, with the snap of the chocolate giving way to the luscious burst of fruit beneath. Savouring chocolate-covered fruits results in a sensual dance between temptation and flavor. The fruit's inherent sweetness is balanced out by the bittersweet embrace of the chocolate, resulting in a delightful flavor interaction that reflects the complexity of desire itself. Partners savor each bite, allowing their taste receptors to act as instruments for a symphony of flavors.

A rich chocolate fondue is a timeless option for a special evening. Place a warm pot of melted chocolate around a variety of fruits, such as strawberries, bananas, and pineapple, as well as marshmallows and bits of pound cake. Encourage your companion to dip these delicious goodies into the decadent pool of chocolate to create intimate and pleasurable shared moments. To create exquisite flavor combinations, chocolate is frequently blended with other ingredients. The meal gains a touch of warmth and sensuality from the way that chile, cinnamon, and cardamom complement the richness of dark chocolate. When chocolate is combined with fruit, such as strawberries or oranges, the sweet and sour flavors are tantalizingly contrasted, arousing the taste buds and resulting in a mellow fusion of experiences. These flavor combinations not only produce a pleasant taste sensation, but they also stimulate desire and eagerness.

Sharing these delectable treasures leads to a shared experience of pleasure and connection. As they share delicious bites with one another, partners look at each other with understanding, creating a climate of caring and affection. The act of feeding and receiving food itself serves as a metaphor for cultivating the emotional ties that link people together. Beyond the physical enjoyment, eating chocolate-covered fruits turns into a nourishing ritual that fosters intimacy. A cocoon of shared luxury is created for couples, where time stands still and the outside world disappears. They can luxuriate in one other's presence in this private haven, strengthening their emotional bond.

Aphrodisiacs have long been used for their arousing effects, which is a testament to the continuing interest with igniting passion through delectable foods. As couples participate in an age-old custom that connects the past and present, exploring these historical strands deepens the experience.

73 | Aldis O. Sherwood

Conclusively, the fusion of chocolate-covered fruits is a tempting tapestry made from the strands of indulgence and desire. The aphrodisiac properties of chocolate and fruits are combined in this delicious adventure, giving couples the chance to partake in an activity that not only piques their palates but also strengthens their bond. In celebration of nature's gifts, lovers explore the sensory worlds of taste and touch as they rekindle their passion and create memories that stay long beyond the last meal. Fruits that have been dipped in chocolate are transformed from simple treats into embodiments of desire, demonstrating the effectiveness of shared indulgence in improving pleasure and establishing close relationships.

CHAPTER EIGHT

Aphrodisiac Drinks - Tempting Libations to Ignite Passion.

It was a bubbling evening; the most entrancing colors of nature were shown. Every building and architectural framework became works of art as the sun set, bathing the surroundings in a warm, golden color. The sound of chirping birds and soft rustling filled the air, giving the impression that nature itself was conversing peacefully. The sky painted itself in hues of pink, orange, and purple as the day slowly faded into the sunset, producing an amazing canvas that seemed to go on forever. The magnificence of nature's show encompassed everyone fortunate enough to view it at this time when the world appeared to pause. It was the evening John and I decided to try the chocolate aphrodisiac drink. The room was filled with an electrifying air of anticipation. The enticing attraction of a chocolate aphrodisiac drink comes to life. An alluring perfume permeates the space, a delicate interplay of velvety cocoa notes blending with the cozy embrace of candlelight. As deep brown velvet drapes fall from the ceiling, they envelop the room in a sumptuous embrace that resembles a secret shared between lovers. The polished mahogany table was covered with porcelain cups, each a beautiful vessel ready for the elixir of desire. The cups contain a chocolate aphrodisiac cocktail that arouses latent senses and unleashes suppressed passions inside their delicate curves, acting as expectant conspirators. Each crystal decanter is holding an elixir of fascination as it stands sentinel. A bowl of smoky chili flakes sits next to a thin, delicate vanilla pod, its blazing intensity a sign of passion. A mound of crushed rose petals sits next to a sprinkle of earthy cinnamon that smells like old rites and is a tribute to ageless passion. The air is filled with a gentle, rhythmic tune that pulses in time with John's accelerated heartbeat and mine. The first sip is an opulent cascade of bittersweet delight that dances across the tongue, teasing and tantalizing with its complexity.

John's eyes and mine meet and their gazes are held in silence speaks volumes about our shared need and scorching intensity. Candlelight creates a ballet of shadows on the walls that mimics the inward dance of feelings and sensations. Our hands roamed each other's bodies, clothes pulled off, and still not getting enough of each other. He tortured me by slowing licking and biting my clit. He swallowed the juices dripping but doesn't want me to reach orgasm. He pulled away and licked his glinting lips. I could see his throbbing dick. Sit up he said. I did as I was told, I was breathless as he kissed down the valley of my breast

Aphrodisiac cocktails emerge as seductive mixtures meant to amuse the senses and stoke sensuality amid the variety of flavors and the attraction of expectation. These enticing libations, steeped in mystery and tradition, enable lovers to explore intimacy like never before by taking them on a captivating trip into a world where taste, fragrance, and desire combine.

Aphrodisiac beverages are more than just libations; they are a symphony of seduction that combines a wide range of flavors and the beauties of nature. This enticing confluence of flavors combines the depth of herbs, the warmth of spices, and the sweetness of fruits to produce a musical fusion that speaks to both the body and the spirit. With a beautiful flavor crescendo, each sip engages the senses like a note in this symphony. Beyond taste, the art of aroma is entwined with the attraction of aphrodisiac beverages. The air is filled with an alluring perfume from the beautiful bouquet of herbs, botanicals, and spices, setting the stage for the upcoming sensory encounter. With each breath, the olfactory senses engage in a seductive ballet that awakens desire and anticipation.

Aphrodisiac beverages are shrouded in mystery because it has long been thought that they might stoke desires. Historical accounts of enticing elixirs and potions of love inspire a sense of magic, linking the past and present. Couples today participate in a contemporary interpretation of these time-honored customs, enjoying the alchemical fusion of tastes to promote intimacy. Drinks with aphrodisiac properties are more than just libations; they are elixirs of intimacy that strengthen relationships between lovers. Making and consuming these libations together turns into a ritualized activity that deepens closeness. Couples experiment with flavors and enjoy the expectation of the aphrodisiac effects as part of the shared experience, which develops a sense of unity and playfulness.

Drinks that are considered to be aphrodisiacs are made with care to kindle the passions of sensuality, heightening the sense of touch and physical sensations. Ginger, which is well recognized for its warming characteristics, and vanilla, which has a calming attraction, are ingredients that help to increase cognition. Couples who indulge in these seductive drinks learn to recognize the intricacies of touch, taste, and emotion. Think about attempting chocolate-based cocktails. A tempting concoction can be made by mixing vodka, cream, raspberry liqueur, and chocolate liqueur. Shake well with ice before straining into a martini glass with a cocoa powder rim. Add a fresh raspberry as a garnish, then watch as your spouse is seduced by the contrasting flavors and textures.

Drinks that are aphrodisiacs are interwoven throughout human history, spanning all eras and cultures. The selection of the fruits, herbs, and spices for their romantic qualities is a monument to the eternal pursuit of intimacy and pleasure. Couples who share in these libations join a long-standing custom that honors the meeting of the abundance of nature and human passion.

As a result, aphrodisiac beverages serve as elixirs of connection, elixirs of intimacy, and potions of desire in addition to being just beverages. These enticing refreshments enable lovers to enjoy in the delights of the senses and set out on a journey of increased sensuality through a fascinating fusion of taste, scent, and tradition. Together, they create moments that transcend the commonplace and fan the flames of love as they embrace the mystique of old knowledge and the modern desire of romance. A toast to desire, a celebration of connection, and a testament to the seductive ability of flavor and aroma to stoke the flames of romance are all made with aphrodisiac beverages.

CHAPTER NINE

Allergies and Dietary Restrictions - Safely Enjoying Chocolate's Benefits.

Consuming chocolate is a widely cherished pleasure, but for people with allergies and dietary limitations, navigating the world of delicacies made with cocoa necessitates striking a delicate balance between enjoyment and caution. It takes a combination of caution, intelligent decision-making, and an unrelenting commitment to enjoying every bite of chocolate without compromising health to safely enjoy its advantages.

A world of potential allergies exists among the appeal of chocolate's decadent flavors, and these need to be carefully considered. Understanding the typical causes, such as nuts, dairy, and soy, which frequently make their way into chocolate formulas, is the first step in a well-informed strategy. Reading labels carefully emerges as a critical skill that enables people to recognize and stay away from chemicals that might cause allergic responses. There are many different chocolate alternatives available because to the innovation that has been sparked by the changing landscape of dietary preferences. Due to its higher cocoa content, dark chocolate frequently represents a dependable option for people who are allergic to dairy. Additionally, a variety of specialist brands now provide chocolates that are nut-free, soy-free, and gluten-free to accommodate a variety of dietary requirements.

Taking control of one's chocolate creations not only enables people but also guarantees a culinary experience that adheres to their nutritional needs. Making homemade chocolates gives chocoholics complete control over the ingredients, allowing them to create delicious confections that are customized to their tastes and allergen sensitivities. This culinary adventure unlocks a world of invention where one's imagination is the only constraint. Examining ingredients is just one aspect of the fight against allergies; cross-contamination is another. The rigorous search for chocolates devoid of allergens could be in vain if the items unintentionally come into contact with allergic substances while being manufactured. Choose products with allergen-free certificates or those produced in settings dedicated to strict cross-contamination prevention measures if you want piece of mind.

A market bursting with allergen-free chocolate substitutes has emerged as a result of the rising tide of dietary restrictions. These specialty products, such as dairy-free bars and nut-free truffles, are geared toward people who want to enjoy themselves without making any sacrifices. Accepting these goods not only provides a risk-free enjoyment but also supports the idea that everyone should enjoy the pleasures of chocolate. Even while chocolate may be enticing, moderation is still the key to indulgent behavior. Even when there are many other options, overindulgence might tip the scales and obscure the possible advantages. Adopting a mindful consumption lifestyle makes sure that the benefits of chocolate easily mesh with general wellbeing.

A crucial component of safe chocolate eating for people with severe sensitivities is getting competent medical advice. A road map for navigating the complex world of allergen management is provided by consulting an allergist and nutritionist, who can also offer tailored dietary advice.

In conclusion, allergies or dietary limitations do not have to quiet the symphony of tastes found in chocolate. People can indulge in the delights of chocolate while preserving their health by arming themselves with knowledge, accepting alternate options, and encouraging a spirit of creative discovery. The journey is characterized by empowerment, adaptation, and the unmistakable claim that enjoyment of chocolate is a fundamental human right, available to everyone who approaches it with prudence, curiosity, and a desire to cherish life's sweet moments.

Moderation And Balance of Chocolate - Understanding the Right Amount For Maximum Pleasure.

The dance of moderation and balance is a timeless truth that exists in the world of indulgence, where cocoa's irresistible seduction dances on the taste buds and caresses the senses. Understanding the perfect amount of chocolate for optimum enjoyment necessitates coordinating a symphony of moderation and appreciation, just as a good conductor leads an orchestra to produce tunes that are harmonic. It is a trip that spans the gap between culinary enjoyment and general wellbeing, delivering a sensory experience that is completely enjoyable, guilt-free, and rewarding.

Think of a square of silky dark chocolate dissolving slowly on the tongue, with each flavor detail unfolding like a subtle note in a captivating tune. The art of savoring takes center stage in order to enhance enjoyment. Each bite turns into a sensory investigation, a request to savor the present and appreciate the subtleties of flavor. This methodical approach turns eating chocolate into a conscious ritual, enhancing the enjoyment and encouraging a strong connection with the experience.

Then, in order to successfully navigate the world of chocolate, balance—the basis of lasting pleasure—becomes the guiding principle. No matter how decadent chocolate may be, finding the appropriate balance is crucial to avoiding overindulgence that can overwhelm its benefits. Similar to how a great tightrope walker maintains balance to cross perilous heights, chocolate lovers too need to find the right balance between delight and excess. In the search for the ideal amount of chocolate, thoughtful consumption emerges as a compass. It entails paying attention to the body's signals, actively participating in the event, and discerning between true desire and intermittent urge.

People can learn to tell when their bodies are craving the joys of chocolate and when they are looking for comfort elsewhere by engaging in mindfulness practices.

The world of chocolate provides a variety of possibilities, including dark, milk, and white, just as an orchestra consists of various instruments that work together to produce a symphony. Each type's nutritional value and advantages differ, which adds another level of complication to the moderation equation. While milk chocolate gives a creamier enjoyment, dark chocolate has antioxidants and possible health advantages. Individuals are better equipped to choose the type that fits their interests and health objectives when they are aware of these little differences.

In conclusion, the struggle to find the ideal chocolate dosage for optimum pleasure is a reflection of the symphony of life itself. It calls for a masterful balancing act of appreciation, control, and a strong bond with the senses. People may master the world of chocolate, reveling in its joys while preserving their wellbeing, by adopting the concepts of savoring, balance, and awareness. This endeavor honors the many facets of chocolate's delights as well as the art of living in complete harmony. It is not just about consumption.

Personal preferences and tolerance for chocolate - tailoring the experience to individuals needs.

The topic of chocolate, a wonderful treat loved by people everywhere, goes beyond taste and includes an ensemble of individual tastes and tolerance levels. In order to create a chocolate experience that deeply resonates with each individual, it is essential to recognize and accommodate these unique variations.

The range of chocolate options, from rich milk chocolate to powerful black cocoa, represents the variety of tastes that exist among people. While some people are drawn to milk chocolate's sweetness, others find comfort in dark chocolate's nuanced bitterness. These personal tastes are not random; rather, a complex interaction of elements including heredity, culture, and individual experiences has an impact on them. Some people are innately more sensitive to the bitterness present in cocoa, and genetic variations lead to disparities in taste perception. Cultural backgrounds also affect what is deemed pleasing because regional flavors and culinary customs develop one's palette.

The chocolate industry has welcomed innovation and personalization in response to these various tastes. For instance, artisanal chocolatiers produce unique concoctions that consider elements like sweetness, bitterness, and texture. Chocolate lovers may now luxuriate in creations made to suit their individual preferences thanks to the emergence of customised packaging and creative taste combinations. Chocolate is now a personalized experience that evokes memories, feelings, and unique preferences rather than just being a generic treat.

Personalization, however, extends beyond just preferences. Chocolate tolerance is a significant factor in how the experience is shaped. Caffeine and theobromine, two substances found in chocolate, have varied effects on different people. While some people might adore these substances, others might feel jittery or restless. Alternatives like dairy-free or sugar-free products are required since allergies and dietary restrictions make things even more difficult.

This comprehension of tolerance served as the inspiration for the development of specialized chocolate goods. Dark chocolate with lower sugar and dairy content is a good choice for people who are concerned about their health. Similar to how chocolates without caffeine or theobromine are marketed to people who are sensitive to stimulants. Today's producers use an integrated approach, making sure that chocolate is not simply a pleasure but also a cozy indulgence that meets everyone's needs.

The complex study of taste and sensory perception further enhances the enjoyment of chocolate. Research explores the nuanced nature of flavor perception, revealing how the olfactory and taste buds work together to produce a complete sensory experience. These skills enable chocolatiers to create chocolates with complex flavors that delight the senses. They produce chocolate that surprises even the most discriminating connoisseurs by experimenting with unusual ingredients and flavor profiles, turning the encounter into a sensory adventure.

The chocolate world is far from being uniform; it is a landscape that is influenced by unique preferences and tolerances. How we experience and enjoy chocolate is influenced by a combination of genetic, cultural, and sensory variables. The chocolate industry makes sure that everyone can enjoy this delicious treat by innovating, customizing, and using scientific findings. Chocolate is more than just a treat; it takes each of us on an expedition of personal taste, comfort, and delight. One thing is certain despite the industry's continued development: different people have different experiences with chocolate.

CHAPTER TEN: CONCLUSION

Summary of Chocolate's Erotic Potential

Sensuality, symbolism, and cultural settings are all woven together in the topic of chocolate's erotic potential to create a seductive experience that arouses pleasure and desire. This delectable dessert is a significant component in the world of romance and intimacy because of its innate capacity to elicit a variety of feelings and sensations.

Chocolate is irresistible because of its decadent texture, alluring flavors, and alluring scent. It's crucial to notice and vividly express these sensory aspects in order to explore its sensual potential. Intimate caresses are symbolized by the velvety texture of chocolate melting on the tongue, and the ecstasy of shared passions is reflected in its decadent flavor. Evocative language that appeals to the reader's senses fosters a deeper comprehension of how chocolate might serve as a vehicle for desire.

Furthermore, chocolate's erotic attraction is further enhanced by the symbolism associated with it. Beyond its culinary allure, chocolate acts as a sentimental gift, expressing feelings that words frequently fall short of. Sharing chocolate is a symbolic act that may be both a lighthearted invitation and a heartfelt declaration of love, fostering a sense of connection that goes beyond simple consumption.

When we take into account chocolate's historical and cultural significance, its erotic potential becomes more complex. Chocolate has long been linked to pleasure, love, and reproduction across cultures and eras. Exploring these cultural differences not only deepens our comprehension but also demonstrates how the attraction of chocolate has stood the test of time, remaining a timeless representation of luxury.

Chocolate's sensuous potential has been embraced in literature and art through sensual allusions and metaphorical depictions. These artistic interpretations highlight the deep influence of chocolate on the human imagination, ranging from literary works that compare the taste of chocolate to a lover's kiss to artwork that depicts chocolate as an embodiment of desire.

Although frequently associated with love relationships, chocolate may also be erotic. Its sensual allure can also be explored through celebrations and self-indulgence. Advertising for chocolate frequently emphasizes the pleasure that can be experienced after eating it. By taking into account these many circumstances, it is clear how chocolate can arouse desire and pleasure in a number of situations.

But it's important to understand that using chocolate as an erotic metaphor might bring up moral dilemmas. Potential hazards include objectification and the maintenance of stereotypes, which serve as a gentle reminder that while chocolate can be a delicious vehicle for desire, it must be treated with respect and sensitivity.

As a result, the intricate combination of sensory perceptions, symbolism, cultural influences, and moral concerns that goes into chocolate's sensual potential is clear. The fact that music may arouse desire, elicit pleasure, and promote connection is proof of its enduring fascination. Chocolate's sensual potential continues to fascinate hearts and stoke passions whether it is shared between lovers, enjoyed alone, or commemorated in cultural traditions, making it a timeless luxury that goes beyond simple confectionery.

Embracing the Sensual Delight of Chocolate in Intimate Connections

The sensuous delights of chocolate provide a gateway to a world where taste, touch, and emotion are

101 | Aldis O. Sherwood

intertwined in close relationships. This mouthwatering delight, acclaimed for its decadent textures and alluring flavors, transforms into an amazing catalyst that arouses desire, strengthens emotional ties, and heightens sensory experiences. To fully appreciate chocolate's alluring function in close relationships, it is crucial to investigate its complex effects in detail and nuance.

The intense engagement of the senses is at the core of this experience. Sharing chocolate takes on a sensory voyage of inquiry and delight that goes beyond the ordinary. When chocolate melts on the tongue, its silky smoothness evokes the seductive caress of a lover, resulting in a complex dance of sensations that titillates and arouses. With each passing second, the anticipation of this sensory delight grows, bridging the distances in both physical and emotional capabilities between partners.

The giving and receiving of chocolate by lovers develops into a powerful ritual that encourages intimacy on numerous levels. Beyond the bites exchanged, it develops into a sharing of vulnerability, a gesture made by both parties to denote trust, openness, and affection. Barriers fall away as each bite is lovingly delivered, allowing a genuine connection to flourish. This shared experience goes beyond the present time and leaves behind memories that last after the chocolate has been enjoyed.

The aphrodisiac properties of chocolate elevate its relevance in close relationships even further. It ideally complements the intimate setting due to the biological reaction it causes, which releases endorphins and serotonin. These "feel-good" hormones improve mood and heighten pleasure, giving the shared experience a greater emotional resonance. The physical and emotional components of a relationship between partners are intertwined as a result of this chemical reaction, which increases the intensity of personal bonds.

Chocolate is used as a metaphor for suppressed feelings. Giving someone a box of chocolates is a sentimental gesture that expresses feelings that are difficult to put into words. Giving involves not only physical luxury but also the rich emotional landscape that supports close relationships. Couples communicate a shared journey and a mutual appreciation of their emotional and physical connections through chocolate.

Although the pleasures of chocolate have been the main topic up to this point, it's important to recognize the ethical considerations that are involved. Sensitivity should be used when using chocolate as a symbol of sensuality in intimate relationships so that it strengthens the link between partners rather than objectifying or dehumanizing people.

Finally, appreciating the sensuous pleasure of chocolate in close relationships goes beyond its flavor and texture. It develops into a private ritual, an emotional exchange, and a sensory experience that goes beyond food. Chocolate is a delicate thread in the tapestry of close relationships, enhancing bonding and forging enduring memories because of the symphony of sensations, emotions, and symbolism woven throughout this experience.